# The Plan Workbook
# Vegetarian/Pescatarian

## *Fall/Winter*

Lyn-Genet Recitas, HHP- Executive Director of Nutrition

## How The Plan Works

The Plan is a method of finding the healthy foods that can cause inflammation, make you overweight and hasten the aging process. Wait- healthy foods make you fat? I know it's counterintuitive, but it's true. Healthy, low calorie foods like green beans, Greek yogurt, salmon, turkey or oatmeal can cause one to two-pound weight gain. Up to 85% of the people that have worked with us at The Plan experience exponential weight gain to these healthy foods.

This doesn't make sense, a calorie in, a calorie out, right? Wrong. Well then how does this happen? The simplest answer is that these foods can trigger an inflammatory response. This inflammatory response triggers a domino effect that ultimately affects your immune system. That "healthy" spinach and egg white omelette may be prematurely aging you, expanding your waistline and cause your health to decline.

What we all need to know is that we are all chemically unique; our weight and our health are just our chemical reactions to food. We also need to remember that aging is a state of inflammation and systems start to slow down as we get older. Our body just can't repair as quickly as it did in our teens and twenties. Digestive enzyme production slows down, stomach acid and saliva decreases all of which aid digestion. Hormonal imbalances trigger yeast flareups which changes our gut flora and our hormones. The foods we used to be able to break down easily when we in our teens and twenties are just harder to break down in our thirties, forties and fifties and beyond.

When you eat a healthy food that doesn't work for

YOUR chemistry there are many systems that are impacted and this inflammatory response can last for 72 hours. Histamine is released, and cortisol levels rise controlling long term fat storage. Increased cortisol production negatively impacts hormones such as progesterone and testosterone.

### The Impact of Cortisol

The more cortisol that is released, the more your hormonal balance is negatively affected. These hormonal fluctuations disrupt water balance, metabolism, thyroid health, healthy sex drive and immune response. Elevated cortisol produces glucose which leads to increased blood sugar levels. Insulin spikes with reactive foods causes yeast to flare. This in turn alters our gut flora. Altered gut flora leads to a weakened immune response as the balance of our intestinal bacteria is thrown off. Remember that 60-70% of our immune system is in our guts! It's a rapid interplay and domino effect that affects our stress levels, moods, health and immune system. And oh, by the way, you're gaining weight...

Wait, isn't it a fact that as you age your metabolism slows down? Well, yes. The thyroid is responsible for your metabolism and the brain only produces 1 teaspoon of thyroid hormone a year. Anything that disrupts a very delicate balance can have long term ramifications. Foods known as goitrogens attack thyroid function and are indicated for exacerbating this underlying condition. Goitrogens include broccoli, spinach, arugula, kale, cabbage, strawberries. Many of the compounds that are present in these foods can become deactivated when cooked. It's ironic that those healthy green juices and raw food diets might be ruining your health, metabolism and your mood.

If you are trying to eat healthfully most of the time, and your health and weight are just not responding, it might be time to find out why your efforts are not paying off as they should. The Plan will help you find *your* path to ultimate health.

## The Role of The Thyroid

The thyroid is a major player when it comes to hormonal health since it stimulates and synchronizes the metabolic cellular functions in every tissue throughout the body.

Thyroid disorders are much more common in women than men until the age of 40. In women, adequate binding of T3 (the active thyroid hormone) is dependent upon sufficient progesterone. A low level of progesterone is a common experience in both young and older women and often contributes to imbalances in thyroid function.

Estrogen levels also strongly impact thyroid function. High levels of estrogen or estrogen dominance lead to high levels of TBG (thyroid binding globulin). TBG binds up all the active thyroid hormones in the blood rendering them useless. So your levels of hormone can appear normal in a blood test but your tissues are not receiving the hormones they should be.

There are certain times in our lives when hormones naturally change (such as postpartum or peri-menopause), making it more likely for estrogen levels to be high and progesterone to be low. So many women have been tested for postpartum depression only to find out that there is no true depression but their thyroid levels are "low". Being labeled as hypothyroid post-partum or during peri-menopause is one thing to really take with a grain of salt since we know that once the estrogen levels come down the thyroid will start functioning again!

Men start to catch up with thyroid imbalances starting in their 40s and by the time they are in their 60s are neck and neck with women at roughly 85% dysfunction. Men who are extreme athletes and vegetarians have a higher rate of thyroid issues and start having imbalances as early as their 20s. Higher rates of stress also affect testosterone and the thyroid in both sexes.

## Common Thyroid Inhibitors

1) Times of extreme hormonal change or stress. Stress will skew testosterone and estrogen.
2) SSRIs- Prozac, Wellbutrin, Zoloft, Celexa etc
3) Hormone therapy
4) Goitrogenic foods (see list on page 8)
5) Overexercise
6) Vegan or vegetarian diets, juice fasts

## Conditions Exacerbated by Low Thyroid Function

1) Energy
2) Sex drive
3) Skin
4) Digestion
5) Migraines
6) Depression
7) Body temperature
8) Hormone balance
9) Sleep

## Thyroid Self-Test:

To test yourself for an under active thyroid:

1. Keep a digital thermometer by your bed at night
2. When you wake up in the morning, place the thermometer in your armpit and hold it there for 2 minutes.
3. Keep still and quiet - any movement of the body can upset your temperature reading and the temperature of the body rises when you begin moving around.
4. A consistent temperature of 97.3°F or lower is indicative of an under active thyroid. I have found when temp is at 96.5 and below the following are affected: energy, weight loss, sex drive, skin health and digestion.

### Natural Ways to Stimulate Thyroid Health

1. Liquid B-12 complex: There are many nutritional deficiencies that account for thyroid dysfunction. B-12 and iodine are two major players in balancing your thyroid function. We recommend these for short term use (2-3 weeks) to bump up your bbt and then taper down once your temperature is consistently in the 96.5 range.
2. Maine Sea Seasonings (available in shaker form) is a wonderful form of iodine, rich in many minerals.
3. Certain animal proteins boost bbt. There is a group of people who respond well to iodine rich foods like cod and scallops and another group who respond better to steak and lamb. Please test the proteins and find which work best for your chemistry.
4. Activities which boost your body temperature are wonderful for increasing thyroid activity- moderate exercise, saunas, hot baths and drinking warm teas all work well.

## Goitrogenic Foods

Goitrogenic foods are compounds that may interfere with thyroid function. Preparation methods, such as cooking or fermentation, reduce the amount of goitrogenic activity in these foods.

As always your chemistry is unique so do not take this list to mean you should not have these foods. It just means that you need to be mindful of how these foods affect you.

**Common goitrogens are**:

- Arugula
- Broccoli- raw
- Broccoli Rabe
- Brussel sprouts
- Cabbage
- Cauliflower
- Collard greens
- Horseradish
- Kale-raw
- Kohlrabi
- Millet
- Mustard
- Peaches
- Peanuts
- Pine nuts
- Radishes
- Raspberries
- Rutabaga
- Soybean and soy products, including tofu and edamame
- Spinach
- Strawberries
- Turnips
- Watercress

**Please remember that eating goitrogenic foods in a raw state is much more problematic for proper thyroid functioning- this includes juicing.**

## Food Sensitivity

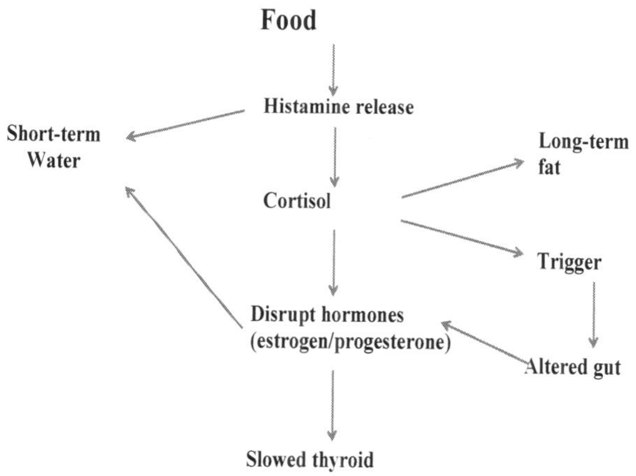

## Introduction to The Plan

### Preparation

You will need:

- A digital scale, which measures in 2/10th of a pound. (We prefer Eatsmart scale with 3.5" LCD screen)
- A digital thermometer
- Liver support — choose from Jarrow or NOW brand Milk Thistle capsules, dandelion tea (any brand you like – we like Yogi Teas), or Herbpharm Healthy Liver Tonic

Please HYDRATE! Your baseline is half your body weight in ounces - the best way to do this is drink a pint all at once. Please drink water in-between meals, not during as drinking during meals can impair your digestion--If you can leave a 45 window before and after each meal that is ideal.

Do *not drink after dinner* and try to finish all water by 7:30 or 3-4 hours before bed. Please do not drink over the recommended water amount as this will affect kidney function and will cause water retention.

### General Guidelines

- Please follow the menus exactly. Do not make substitutions or changes without prior approval.
- Do not swap lunch and dinner from different days. Ex: day 5 lunch with day 4 dinner. Do not have soup for dinner if you switch lunch and dinner, you can have steamed or sautéed vegetables instead to aid digestion of raw vegetables.

- Please start each day with 16 oz of water and fresh lemon juice plus your liver support of choice (See the Preparation section above)
- Many clients ask about eating out and we discourage this in the first ten days because too much of weight gain comes from excess sodium and a meal prepared in a restaurant can have 3 days worth of sodium! This is why we ask that you please set aside 8-10 days in the beginning of your plan to prepare your meals at home. This will ultimately decrease weight gain from travel and eating out.

**Days 1 to 4**

- Do not work out the first three days. This is detox time when the body is repairing your organs. If you work out during this time, energy is spent on muscle repair instead of repairing vital organs. You have the rest of your life to work out. RELAX! I have found that weight loss increases if you do not work out the first three days and if you limit working out to four times a week. The least inflammatory forms of exercise if you are conditioned are running for a half hour, weight training for 30-45 minutes and yoga. The types of exercise that are the most problematic are bootcamp, crossfit, Bikram and spinning.
- Your energy level should be fine. However, if you feel tired, this is an indication that the body has a lot of repair to do. When the body gets a break from digesting carbs, animal protein and dairy, the first thing it wants to do is start repairing whatever is damaged in the body. It's during periods of sleep that the body does its best homeostatic work (see Sleep and Repair below).

- Use only lemon juice and extra-virgin olive oil for salad dressing, unless otherwise indicated
- No vinegar until Day 4
- No coffee until after Day 4 (If you think you are going to get a headache, drink black tea with silk coconut milk— up to 2 cups). While coffee is a good anti-oxidant, it is mildly stressful to the liver. We are looking to boost liver health during the cleanse, which will increase weight loss.

## Water

Water is responsible for every metabolic process. If you are dehydrated, you run the risk of exacerbating reactive weight gain, kick starting chronic or latent health issues PLUS you are prematurely aging yourself.

- If you drink less than two glasses of your recommended daily water intake, you will retain .5 lbs of water weight.

Do NOT "overload" your body at the end of the day to make up what you didn't drink earlier. This can overload your kidneys and will most likely show up as water retention the next morning. For the same reason, please drink your last pint of water before your dinner. If at all possible finish water by 7:00 pm or 4 hours before you go to bed. If you drink water after dinner it will hamper digestion and show up as weight gain.

The lower your weight, the less water intake you require. As you lose weight, refer back to the calculator to ensure you're on track.

## Reactions

Reactive response can be anywhere from .5 to 4 lbs. As a general rule of thumb: the amount of weight gain indicates the amount of reactivity. When you are reactive to a food, it can take up to 72 hours for normal functioning to resume. This will include weight loss, normal bowel movements, return of digestive functioning, and a decrease in your genetic "maladies." Taking a probiotic after a reactive food will help you regain normal functioning sooner.

## Weight Plateaus

When you lose weight quickly, you may hit a plateau. This is a natural reaction as your body adjusts to the new weight. Plateaus occur because in prehistoric times the body needed to defend itself in case the weight loss was due to lack of food and possible starvation.

Keep eating according to The Plan. Do not lower food intake. The body will see that food is still coming in, determine there is no fear of starvation and weight loss will resume.

## Sleep and Repair

When we do not get enough sleep, our organs do not have adequate time to do the repair and restoration that is so vital to our health. This actually contributes to higher acid levels in the cells and increased inflammation. High acidity and inflammation are markers for weight gain and slowed weight loss.

## Food Tips

### Coffee

- After Day 3 you may drink 1 cup of coffee per day with half and half and the sweetener of your choice. Your choice of sweeteners is agave and honey. If you don't have those then brown or white sugar is fine. Please do not have any other sweetener including stevia.

### Salt

- No salt until after Day 4. After Day 4, sea salt may be used in moderation. You will find that after the cleanse, your taste for salt will have decreased significantly.
- We use the Heart Association's guidelines of 1500 mg of sodium per day. Sea salt (as opposed to table salt and kosher salt) has 80 minerals, which help to metabolize the sodium.
- Maine Sea Seasonings (available at Amazon.com) is wonderful salt alternative especially if you suffer from hypothyroidism. These seasonings are made from seaweed and are rich in minerals.

### Dairy

- Please choose full-fat milk when you test. Second best choice is low-fat. Do not use non-fat or skim milk products. Research indicates that the rise in Type 2 Diabetes is due to consumption of reduced-fat dairy products. Until you test milk, please have half and half with your coffee.
- Goat and sheep milk products are much easier to digest than cow's milk. You will be tested on these cheeses first. There are many types of goat and sheep cheese — from gouda to cheddar. They are all acceptable for testing.

- Do NOT have feta or blue cheese during The Plan due to high sodium and/or mold content.

**General Food Guidelines**

- Grains — Brown rice and basmati rice are both excellent low reactive grains. Brown rice is more nutritious, while basmati rice is easier on digestion. Due to high arsenic levels we are recommending that you use basmati rice if at all possible.
- Nuts — Choose only raw, unsalted nuts. NO roasted nuts until you test them. Men should have 1.5 oz as their serving (a large handful), women should have 1 oz (a large handful).

**Oils**

- Cooking at high temperatures can damage oils. The more Omega-3 fatty acids in the oil, the less suitable it is for cooking. Heat not only damages the fatty acids, it can also change them into harmful substances.
- Olive oil and grapeseed oil are best for cooking as long as you do not heat it above its smoke point. This is very important, especially to people who are ill or over the age of 40. Limit use of grapeseed oil as it is higher in omega 6 (the pro-inflammatory oil)
- To preserve the nutritious properties and flavor of unrefined oils, try the "wet-sauté," a technique practiced by gourmet chefs: Pour around one-fourth of a cup of water in to a stir fry pan and heat just below boiling. Then add the food and cook it a bit before adding the oil. Wet-sauté shortens the time an oil is in contact with a hot pan.
- It is fine to add butter once a day, but please do not sauté with butter or cook at high heat.

- Days 4 and forward: A simple vinaigrette is great if you don't have yeast, please do not use mustard. If you suspect yeast is an issue stay with the Lime Agave Vinaigrette in your cookbook.

**Wine**

- Wine is WONDERFUL in moderation. It enhances digestion, is a mild diuretic and decreases stress. One glass of red wine is allowed beginning on Day 4. Do not consume white wine as it is more acidic and will slow weight loss. Wine is allowed after dinner as it aids digestion and decreases cortisol.

**Snacks, Substitutions**

- You may always replace a snack that is mentioned with ½ piece of approved fruit and nuts/seeds.
- You may always replace hummus with 2 tbsp raw almond butter or ½ piece of fruit and pumpkin/sunflower seeds.
- You can always replace soup with steamed or sautéed veggies of any approved vegetables.

**Useful kitchen implements to have on hand:**

- Sharp knives
- Cutting boards
- A salad spinner
- Large sauté pan
- Citrus zester
- Measuring cups + spoons

## Frequently Asked Questions

*Should I stop my medications when I start The Plan?*

While we do often find that medications can be cut down dramatically once you get started, please make sure to discuss with your doctor before you discontinue or taper down any medication.

*Can I do The Plan if I'm breastfeeding?*

For moms still breastfeeding, The Plan works beautifully, but should only be done under the care of one of our staff because the weight loss on The Plan is very rapid and we may need to adjust variables so that it does affect breast milk supply.

*If I have diabetes do I need a specific menu?*

We have found that diabetics do beautifully on The Plan using regular or thyroid menus – no specific menu is needed. Sugars often stabilize within the first 2-3 days for both type 1 and type 2 diabetics, so we recommend being in contact with your doctor to lower oral medications or insulin dosages as needed.

*I'm under 35, can I still do The Plan?*

Yes! Doing The Plan under age 35 is still very valuable to improve health. For clients that are under 35 and have a chronic health condition (eczema, migraines, diabetes, etc.) weight is still a very accurate gauge. However, we have found that weight is not as accurate of a gauge of reactivity for those under 35 who don't have a chronic health condition, we recommend paying attention to the physical cues (gas/bloating, constipation/diarrhea, headaches, fatigue) as indications to discovering your reactive foods.

*I'm doing The Plan for health reasons, but don't want to lose any more weight?*

We work with many clients who want to improve their health but do not need to lose weight. We have found that during the cleanse you may still lose a small amount of weight as the body lets go of inflammation, but the body will quickly find its natural set point where weight will stabilize. At this point, you can judge reactivity by seeing weight go up and a friendly day will be where the weight stays at your set point.

*I'm concerned that I have a health issue that would prevent me from doing The Plan. How do I find out?*

The Plan can work for everybody (that's the beauty of a program that's about *your* individual chemistry!). However there are some conditions, such as diverticulitis, where we do prefer that you work directly with a nutritionist to monitor progress. If you aren't sure what is best in your particular situation, please email info@lyngenet.com to inquire.

*How does a woman's monthly cycle impact testing and reactivity?*

Many women find that their weight stabilizes/goes up and their reactive response is amplified the 2-3 days prior to their cycle because of hormone-related water retention. Let's say a food, i.e.: fish is really only mildly reactive to you and normally cause you to stabilize, if you're PMSing, it can amplify that reactive response a .5 - 1 lb. gain. Every woman is different with the amount of gain they see and for how long, so make sure to pay attention to your cycles before you start The Plan to have a sense of how your body typically responds! As you continue on The Plan, hormone balance dramatically improves, so every month you are on The Plan, you will see less water retention and fewer PMS symptoms prior to your cycle.

A good rule of thumb for most women is to avoid testing new foods (stick with friendly days) the 2-3 days prior to your cycle to prevent an exacerbated reactive response. If you notice PMS for a week before your cycle, rotate in a week of friendly day menus for the best results. Once you start your period and feel good, you can pick right back up with testing and collecting your data.

*What can I expect during detox? What medications are safe to take for a detox headache?*

We have devised the detox to be as easy as possible (no juice fasts or master cleanse here!), but sometimes toxic buildup can cause some discomfort. It is better to deal with this now rather than later on when disease starts to crop up in a more serious form. Try double strength peppermint tea to help with nausea. If you have a headache and aspirin is part of your protocol, we have found Excedrin Migraine or Bayer to work very well!

*I am worried that I might be hungry, especially during the cleanse?*

Not at all! In fact, we often have clients who can't finish every meal. Our goal is to chemically balance all meals and have you eat until you feel full so that you feel completely satisfied. In fact, on the first day of the

CLEANSE, you are consuming 2600 calories with 78 grams of protein and 80 grams of fiber.

*Is there an alternative to the Flax Granola?*

Until you test more foods, you can substitute the Blueberry Pear Compote or the smoothie. It will not have the exact same digestive benefits as the flax and some people find it less filling. Please add sunflower seeds as a topping to the compote. The recipe can be found in our menus.

## WATER QUESTIONS

*Does the Dandelion tea get counted as part of my water intake?*

Yes, the Dandelion tea that you drink in the morning as your liver tonic does get counted towards your water intake.

*What else can I drink besides water?*

Peppermint tea, Chamomile tea, and Rooibos teas are all fine to have included as part of your water intake. You may also have Green or Black teas, but I would limit those to 16 oz. daily because of their acidity.

*Why can't you drink with meals?*

Drinking water with meals dilutes digestive enzymes, which will impair digestion. It also causes you to be prematurely full and we want you to fill up on food so that you aren't hungry in an hour or two! It is best to wait 45 minutes before and after your meals to have water.

*Does coffee count as part of my water intake when I include it starting on day 4?*

Coffee does not count towards your daily water total.

*Should I add extra water for wine and when is it best to have wine?*

Yes! It's best to add an extra 4-5 oz. to your daily total for every glass of wine you have and it's good to include that water earlier in the day (before 7:30 pm). You can have wine later at night (up until bedtime!).

*What can I do if I am drinking all of my water but am still thirsty?*

I would first make sure that you added in any extra water that you might need for wine or exercise. If you are still thirsty at this point then please try adding lemon juice to your water. The extra vitamin C helps the cells of the body to absorb and use the water more efficiently, so you will feel less thirsty.

*When do I need to stop drinking water?*

While eating after 7:30 is fine, for optimal digestion and weight data it is critical not to drink water with or after dinner and at least 4 hours before bed.

*How do I adjust my water intake for exercise?*

A good rule of thumb is to add in 8 oz. for every 30 minutes of exercise. You may drink less or more according to thirst. Keep exercise to 20 minutes the first 10-14 days for best results. Intense exercise may slow weight loss.

*How do I adjust water intake for hot weather?*

In hot weather, make adjustments similar to exercise (one or two additional glasses depending upon the severity of the heat, how much time you spend outdoors, etc.). This is especially important for those of you who get migraines because heat can dehydrate you and trigger migraines. Staying out in the heat too long can start to cause your body to overheat and impair your lymphatic system. We see this especially when gardening outdoors for hours. It is best to take breaks from the heat by going inside and cooling off every 30 minutes if possible. You may notice weight stabilization in the next day.

## THYROID QUESTIONS

*My basal body temperatures range between 96.3 and 96.7 – do I need to take the Kelp and B12 supplements?*

If your temperatures are above 96 then just get started with a thyroid-friendly menu and it should work to increase your temperature beautifully. If your temperatures are below 96 after the first 10 days, then you may wish to try adding in these supplements and see if they help. If they do not you may wish to book a consultation.

*Which Maine Coast Sea Seasonings should I purchase?*

The Kelp or Dulse shaker varieties work best.

*I'm on thyroid medication – do I still need to do the thyroid test?*

Yes, it's important to see how the medication is working at the tissue level. If the temperatures are 96 or below, adding in the supplements should help to support the medication.

## Supplements

### Methylsulfonylmethane (MSM)

### MSM and Allergies

MSM helps to alleviate the symptoms of a large number of allergies including food allergies, contact allergies, inhalation allergies, etc. The major anti-allergic property of MSM is caused by its ability to bind to the mucosa and present a natural blocking interface between hosts and allergens

### What do we use MSM for at The Plan?

- Acid Reflux
- Allergies- food and environmental
- Arthritis
- Asthma
- Healthy collagen synthesis - skin, hair, nails and joints
- Inflammation (especially of mucous membranes)
- Leaky gut

### How do I take MSM?

Therapeutic dosage is 3,000-6,000 mg and long term change has been seen after 6 weeks of usage. Noticeable results are usually seen within 2 to 21 days (certain problems may take much longer to notice changes)

### SAM-e

SAM-e stands for S-adenosyl methionine and is made in the body from a reaction between methionine, an amino acid and adenosine triphosphate. SAM-e is involved in many different reactions in the body and levels drop as we age. It has been used to treat depression, hormonal imbalance, liver problems, joint pain, fibromyalgia, and arthritis. It has been shown to increase serotonin. Sam-e is contraindicated for bi-polar disorder and may interfere with Parkinsons' medications.

At The Plan we have found that SAM-e's ability to mitigate the stress response has allowed our clients to have better weight loss in stressful times.

**Probiotics**

A lot of our clients start The Plan with a long history of digestive discomfort. We see clients with everything from incredibly serious Crohn's and Colitis to frustrating and persistent constipation, gas and bloating. Probiotics are one of the things we have found that can really speed up healing and progress on The Plan for clients with these histories.

When many of us think of bacteria, we think of the bad bacteria (strep, e.coli, etc) that causes us to feel sick. But the reality of it is, our digestive tract is filled with trillions of bacteria and much of it is (and should be) good bacteria. In fact, scientists estimate that the bacteria populating our system weighs up to 5 lbs!! This bacterium makes up its own microbiome in our bodies and has a wide range of impacts on our health. When the balance of bacteria is healthy (yeast and bad bacteria are not overwhelming the good guys) it helps to regulate our hormonal systems and our immune systems. That's right--our gut flora plays a huge impact on how often we get sick and how our body is able to fight off infections of all types (including urinary infections and respiratory infections). When the balance of flora in the body gets disrupted it can cause diarrhea, gas, bloating, food cravings, yeast infections, and an increase in colds and flu's. Recent research has also found that disrupted microflora in the body is also heavily implicated in the development of autoimmune diseases.

On The Plan, we have found that starting clients during the detox on a multi-strain probiotic helps to restore the balance of flora in the body more quickly. While Planning you are giving good bacteria the fuel they need to create a healthy digestive tract. Starting on probiotics ensures that you crowd out any bad bacteria at the same time. For clients with a history of digestive issues or impaired immunity they may find that taking probiotics for a week or longer at first will help to speed up the healing dramatically. For clients without any previous health issues, we recommend using the probiotics only as needed after a reactive response to help the body return to balance more quickly.

**Overtraining Can Slow Weight Loss and Repair**

Experience with thousands of clients at The Plan has shown us that over-training not only impedes weight loss but can also cause weight gain — it's nice to see that studies are starting to back us up!

Exercise tends to be pro-inflammatory when it is done for an extended period of time and when there is extended periods of elevated heart rate with no decrease in heart rate. Simply taking breaks and allowing your heart rate to decrease to a normal resting level can make all the difference!

We have been compiling information for over 7 years and have found that:

- Women and men over the age of 40 who exercise 5-6 days a week lose 25% less weight than those who exercise 3-4 times a week.

- People who exercised every other day had the best results for weight loss.
- Exercising for more than 30-45 min (depending on the exercise) slowed weight loss or caused weight gain.
- The biggest culprits are bootcamp, crossfit style classes, Bikram and spinning.

While people may be tempted to say that this weight gain could be attributed to building muscle, we have found that the days where there is weight gain from exercise there is also a corresponding aggravation of people's health issues, and bbt drops. Insulin may rise as well as blood pressure. This indicates the exercise is affecting much more than hypertrophy and muscle repair and is inflammatory.

Over-training has been shown to decrease blood levels of l-glutamine, dopamine and 5-HTP which affect mood, energy and the body's ability to repair. Excessive exercise can negatively affect the hypothalamus and pituitary both of which can lead to or exacerbate thyroid dysfunction. Once you affect the thyroid you are hitting a master gland that regulates everything from your energy levels, mood, sex drive, hormonal response and ability to lose weight (to just name a few of the functions!). In addition, overexercising will increase cortisol levels which increases insulin output and encourages fat storage. In fact, cortisol can *suppress* metabolic activity to preserve energy. The increase in cortisol depletes progesterone or testosterone levels creating estrogen dominance; another reason for weight gain and thyroid dysfunction. Exercising for more than half an hour has been shown to increase hunger thus often offsetting the metabolic boost and calorie burning activity, creating a calorie surplus- not a deficit.

In addition, as we age the body's ability to withstand oxidative stress diminishes. Periods of constantly elevated heart rate with no decrease seems to cause the most damage. Not allowing for adequate periods of rest after oxidative stress heightens inflammation.

If you are gaining weight from exercise or your bbt is dropping then it is PRO-inflammatory for you....meaning it is going to interfere with weight loss efforts, accelerate aging and trigger health issues. In order to avoid health and weight frustrations, we encourage our clients to "test" their favorite exercise as a health variable to see exactly how it affects their body.

**Why am I gaining so much weight eating gluten free?**

Many people are now aware of how much damage foods can do to your digestion and ultimately your health; remember that 70% of your immune system is in your digestive tract! Eating anything daily can build a food sensitivity and our motto at The Plan is "Rotate or React!" Eating foods that have extra gluten added to flour will exacerbate any underlying digestive issues. These foods can include bagels, pasta and pizza dough. But there is hope! Fresh pasta dough usually uses lighter flour and thin crust pizza often contains less gluten as well. Remember you should never feel bloated after a meal so if you do that's a sign from your body saying, "please don't feed this to me!"

While many people may believe they have gluten intolerance (and many that have been on The Plan have realized they don't) gluten free products can be just as problematic. The alternate grains used are often reactive and will continue to affect digestion and weight in a negative fashion.

Unfortunately, a big player in gluten free bread is tapioca starch and potato starch. Tapioca is highly inflammatory and has a glycemic index of 94. Now when you consider that our daily intake should be 100 you can see why weight gain can be a problem if this is the major ingredient! Potato starch has been linked to various disorders such as arthritis, eczema, psoriasis and fibromyalgia. We know that when foods trigger inflammatory diseases an uptick on the scale always follows. In fact, it's the starch of the potato that causes the most weight gain.

Our work on The Plan has found quinoa to be 60% reactive. Teff, which is often used as well, will most likely fall under the same category of inflammation. Why is this? The body is pretty amazing at streamlining operations. If a grain isn't around for a few thousand years the body will often lose the enzymes to break it down. Please consider this before jumping on the latest ancient grain bandwagon. The body also responds best to what has been part of your genetic past- teff is from Ethiopia and quinoa from the Andes- naturally if you are from either of these regions you have a better chance of digesting these grains. Please make sure to rinse quinoa thoroughly; the saponins in quinoa can cause eye and respiratory issues as well as GI distress.

Xanthan gum which is a thickening agent is often used and it is high in purines which affect uric acid levels and this can aggravate pain and inflammation. This is especially noted for people with gout.

Corn has been 80% reactive with my clients and it is often GMO modified. Even if you buy organic corn, GMO may still be a problem. Experts fear that cross-pollination has already begun with GMO corn as the pollen grains are among the largest and heaviest of wind-pollinated plants. I often see clients gain a pound from the simple pleasure of a summer corn on the cob.

So what does this mean if you can't tolerate gluten? That you shouldn't have any sort of bread at all? That's not the purpose of this information - really I'm not here to torture you! What I DO want you to know is that if you find your body is not responding the way it should then GF might be the problem. Try to avoid having daily ingestion of these products and give your body a chance to rest and decrease inflammatory response. We have found rice flour, coconut flour and almond flour to be the most easily digested; when looking at labels make sure that this is the primary ingredient. Please avoid brown rice flour products as the arsenic content is much higher. It's also important to remember that just because something is pro-inflammatory for a certain population, does NOT mean it's going to be a problem for you. Just listen to your body- it will tell you everything you need to know!

## Plan Guidelines

**Beet carrot salad**- grate 4-5 carrots and 1 small beet. Should make 4 servings- stores well in Tupperware

**Portions-** *Unless portions are noted please eat until you are full.*

- Manchego or Sheep's milk parmesan (pecorino Romano): 1-2 tbsp per serving
- Goat's cheese: 1 oz
- Please do not exceed 1.5 oz daily of cheese
- Nuts: unless noted is a handful, which is roughly 1 oz

**Carrot ginger soup-** our anti-inflammatory soup which freezes very well and is very friendly when added to lunch after a reactive day.

**Snacks-** you may always replace snack that is mentioned with a ½ piece of fruit and nuts. You may also always replace hummus with raw almond butter or fruit with pumpkin/sunflower seeds.

**Dessert-** can be 1 oz chocolate or microwaved ½ piece of fruit with cinnamon (pear, apple or ½ cup berries with cinnamon). Limit chocolate to 1 oz daily.

**Butter-** you can add it in once a day, but please do not sauté with butter.

**EVO**- You should be consuming 3-5 tbsp of extra virgin olive oil a day. **Why is EVO so important?** The brain is 60% fat so we need good fats for cognitive functioning. Our cell walls have a phospholipid barrier to we need fat for immune function- evo is an omega 9 so it acts as a catalyst for anti-inflammatory omega 3 (present in your flax, chia and hemp seeds) and fat keeps you full longer!

Please HYDRATE! Your baseline is half your body weight in ounces - the best way to do this is drink a pint all at once. Please drink water in-between meals, not during as drinking during meals can impair your digestion-- if you can leave a 45 window before and after each meal that is ideal. Do not drink after dinner and try to finish all water intake by 7:30 or 3-4 hours before bed. Please do not drink over the recommended water amount as this will affect kidney function and will cause water retention.

## General Protein, Food and Testing Information

*For more information on general plan guidelines please reference the Intro to The Plan.*

## Protein Ranges

- Breakfast — 10-40 grams of protein
- Lunch — 15-25 grams of protein **(stay with 15 grams unless you are an athlete)**
- Dinner — 25-60 grams of protein

## Dense Food Guidelines

- 1 dense grain carbohydrate a day MAX (rice or bread)
- 1 animal protein a day MAX
- 1 bean a day MAX

*If you want to try more than one serving of these per day you can plug a larger portion in for a test day!*

## Combination Tests

Combining animal protein, grain or legumes together at the same meal is a test. Example: rice (grain) and fish (animal protein) or bread (grain) and eggs (animal protein). Coconut Milk and animal proteins is a test as well.

## Good Low Reactive Sources of Protein: Aim for 15-25 grams of protein for lunch

**Broccoli-** 5 grams per cup
**Sunflower seeds-** 5 grams per oz (these two are also good sources of calcium!)
**Pumpkin seeds-** 9 grams per oz (great source of zinc for your immune system!)
**Almonds-** 8 grams per oz

**Cheese-** 8 grams per oz
**Chickpeas-** 5 grams per 1/2 cup
**Rice** – 6 grams per 1 cup
**Chia-** 5 grams per 2 tbsp (A great source of omega-3's!)
**Hemp Seed** – 11 grams per 3 tbsp (great for iron, magnesium, potassium and zinc)

**Winter Menus**

In winter we always have either a cooked vegetable or a soup with lunch to aid digestion. Dinner always has cooked vegetables and a raw vegetable salad as raw vegetables contain enzymes.

**Approved Salad Greens**

Approved salad greens for fall/winter are baby romaine, red leaf lettuces, Boston lettuce, frisée, escarole, dandelion. Any mixed greens blend that has arugula, watercress, tat soi or spinach is a test. Colder vegetables like Romaine hearts and cucumbers may cause gas and bloating. If they do, immediately take a probiotic and discontinue use. They will cause weight gain and digestive issues. For animal protein it is best to stay with baby romaine as your lettuce greens of choice. Your salad dressing for the first 3 days is lemon juice, extra virgin olive oil and herbs of choice (ex: dill, tarragon, basil).

## Women's Vegetarian/Pescatarian Days 1-20

### Day One

### Breakfast

1 cup Flax granola with ½ cup blueberries or ½ pear
Silk Coconut milk or Rice Dream- this will be your breakfast "milk" until you test a new milk

### Lunch

Carrot ginger soup – with sunflower seeds
2 cups sautéed or steamed broccoli
Baby Romaine

### Snack

1 apple

### Dinner

Sautéed kale, 3-4 carrots, onion, zucchini, shiitakes, and broccoli with spicy coco sauce Grated Carrot and raw grated beet salad with pumpkin seeds-
**Quick and easy version: make the spicy coco sauce, add all the vegetables to it and let it simmer for 10 minutes.**

| | | |
|---|---|---|
| Health goals for next 20 days | | |
| | | |
| Long term health goals | | |
| | | |
| Weight goal short term | | Long term |
| Weight | Bbt | Water day prior |
| Hrs slept | Exercise | |

## Day Two

### Breakfast
Flax with ½ cup blueberries or ½ apple

### Lunch
Carrot ginger soup with sunflower seeds
Baby Romaine with ¼ avocado, lemon and evo
2 cups sautéed or steamed broccoli

### Snack
1 pear with 8 almonds

### Dinner
Leftover sautéed kale and veggies
1 cup basmati rice with pumpkin seeds
beet/carrot salad with sunflower seeds

| | | |
|---|---|---|
| Weight | Bbt | Water day prior |
| Hrs slept | Stress level 1-10 | |
| Menu switches | | |
| Exercise- intensity/duration | | |
| Health- symptoms | | |
| Digestion | | |

## Day Three: Lentils

### Breakfast
Flax with choice of ½ cup blueberries or ½ pear

### Lunch
Baby romaine with ¼ avocado, carrots & pumpkin seeds
Cream of Broccoli soup

### Snack
12-15 almonds

### Dinner
1 cup of lentils on a bed of baby romaine with sunflower seeds
Oven roasted zucchini, broccoli, carrots, onions, garlic and Italian herb blend- finish with orange oil and fresh black pepper

| | | |
|---|---|---|
| Weight | Bbt | Water day prior |
| Hrs slept | Stress level 1-10 | |
| Menu switches | | |
| Exercise- intensity/duration | | |
| Health- symptoms | | |
| Digestion | | |

**Day Four: Cheese** *(you may now have one cup of coffee in the morning, homemade vinaigrette and wine at night with or after dinner. Please do not consume any water with or after dinner)*

**Breakfast**
Flax Granola with ½ cup berries, ½ apple or ½ pear

**Lunch**
Leftover roasted vegetables (reheat) on a bed of baby romaine with pumpkin seeds and 1 oz goat cheese (hard or soft)

**Snack**
Carrots with 2 tbsp raw almond butter
or
1/8th cup sunflower seeds and 1 tbsp dried cranberries (Plan Trail Mix)

**Dinner**
Rice salad—warm with sunflower seeds and pumpkin seeds
Sautéed broccoli and zucchini
Radicchio and pomegranate salad

| | | |
|---|---|---|
| Weight | Bbt | Water day prior |
| Hrs slept | Stress level 1-10 | |
| Menu switches | | |
| Exercise- intensity/duration | | |
| Health- symptoms | | |
| Digestion | | |

**Day Five**: **Test New Protein** *(you may now have sea salt & dessert nightly)*

**Breakfast**

Blueberry pear compote
Or
Apple Streusel

**Lunch**

Baby Romaine w/carrot/beet/radicchio salad & sunflower seeds
Cream of Broccoli soup

**Snack**

Plan Trail mix
Or
Apple chips with almonds

**Dinner**

Test a new protein (scallops, chickpeas, egg whites) on a bed of baby romaine or frisée
Sautéed or grilled zucchini with onion and basil finished pumpkin seeds and goat cheese

| | | |
|---|---|---|
| Weight | Bbt | Water day prior |
| Hrs slept | Stress level 1-10 | |
| Menu switches | | |
| Exercise- intensity/duration | | |
| Health- symptoms | | |
| Digestion | | |

**Day Six**: **No test**

**Breakfast**
Flax with choice of ½ cup berries, ½ apple or ½ pear
Or
Apple Streusel

**Lunch**
Baby romaine with radicchio apple, ¼ avocado, pumpkin seeds
Steamed Broccoli with lemon and evo

**Snack**
Zucchini noush
Or
Apple chips (*Bare Fruit* is a great brand and can be ordered online or bought at Costco)

**Dinner**

Any approved protein
Warm kale salad with sunflower seeds
Carrot/beet salad

| | | |
|---|---|---|
| Weight | Bbt | Water day prior |
| Hrs slept | Stress level 1-10 | |
| Menu switches | | |
| Exercise- intensity/duration | | |
| Health- symptoms | | |
| Digestion | | |

## Day Seven: Optional test hemp seeds
## Breakfast

Blueberry Pear Compote
Or
Flax granola with ½ cup blueberries, ½ apple or ½ pear

### Lunch
Leftover warm kale salad with pumpkin seeds

Baby romaine with grated carrots, sunflower seeds or 2 tbsp hemp seeds (if testing)

### Snack
Zucchini noush with apple chips
Or
Apple chips and almonds

### Dinner
Any approved protein on a bed of baby romaine or frisée
Sautéed vegetables- broccoli, carrots, zucchini, onions

| | | |
|---|---|---|
| Weight | Bbt | Water day prior |
| Hrs slept | Stress level 1-10 | |
| Menu switches | | |
| Exercise- intensity/duration | | |
| Health- symptoms | | |
| Digestion | | |

## Day Eight: Optional test new protein

### Breakfast
Blueberry Pear Compote
Or
Flax granola cereal with ½ piece approved fruit

### Lunch
Leftover Sautéed vegetables on a bed of salad of choice with sunflower seeds and almond slivers
Optional: Basil escarole soup

### Snack
Plan Trail Mix

### Dinner
Protein that has been tested –make sure to rotate
OR
Test a new protein
Roasted, Sautéed, Grilled or steamed vegetables that have been approved with 2 tbsp grated manchego
Radicchio and 1/8th cup pomegranate arils or ¼ apple

| | | |
|---|---|---|
| Weight | Bbt | Water day prior |
| Hrs slept | Stress level 1-10 | |
| Menu switches | | |
| Exercise- intensity/duration | | |
| Health- symptoms | | |
| Digestion | | |

## Day Nine: Optional Test New Cereal

### Breakfast

Blueberry pear compote
Or
Test new cereal (arrowhead mills rice and shine, rice flakes or spelt flake cereals are a good place to start. Rice is the safest choice). Add 2 tbsp chia and sunflower seeds and approved fruit

### Lunch

Baby Romaine with leftover vegetables (reheated), pumpkin seeds, ¼ avocado and goat cheese
Or
Omit goat cheese and add ½ cup low sodium chickpeas or 2 tbsp hemp seeds (choose one)

### Snack

½ piece of fruit and almonds
Or
Zucchini noush with apple chips

### Dinner

Any approved protein
Carrot/beet/radicchio salad
Sautéed broccoli, shiitakis, carrots and garlic

| | | |
|---|---|---|
| Weight | Bbt | Water day prior |
| Hrs slept | Stress level 1-10 | |
| Menu switches | | |
| Exercise- intensity/duration | | |
| Health- symptoms | | |
| Digestion | | |

## Day Ten: Test new protein

### Breakfast
Any Approved Breakfast

### Lunch
Baby romaine or red leaf lettuce, carrots and pumpkin seeds
Cream of Broccoli Soup

### Snack
Apple chips
Or
½ piece of fruit and almonds

### Dinner
Test New Protein (Grilled ***wild*** white fish, chickpeas, scallops, lentils, tempeh or pinto beans
Sautéed kale and with sunflower seeds, avocado
Radicchio and pomegranate salad (or apple)

| | | |
|---|---|---|
| Weight | Bbt | Water day prior |
| Hrs slept | Stress level 1-10 | |
| Menu switches | | |
| Exercise- intensity/duration | | |
| Health- symptoms | | |
| Digestion | | |

## Day Eleven: No test

### Breakfast
Apple Streusel
Or
Previously tested approved Cereal with chia seeds, sunflower seeds and approved fruit

### Lunch
Leftover sautéed kale with carrots, avocado and pumpkin seeds
Optional: Basil escarole soup

### Snack
Katie's Kale Chips
Or
Plan Trail mix

### Dinner
Any approved protein
Sautéed approved vegetables with lime and garlic
Salad of choice with sunflower seeds

| | | |
|---|---|---|
| Weight | Bbt | Water day prior |
| Hrs slept | Stress level 1-10 | |
| Menu switches | | |
| Exercise- intensity/duration | | |
| Health- symptoms | | |
| Digestion | | |

## Day Twelve: Test new vegetable

### Breakfast
Blueberry pear compote
Or
Apple Streusel
Or
Smoothie

### Lunch
Leftover vegetables reheated with goat cheese
Carrots with raw almond butter

### Snack
Katie's Kale Chips
Or
Apple chips
Or
Carrots with 2-3 tbsp hummus (only if you have tested)

### Dinner
Approved protein on a bed of baby romaine or frisée
Test new vegetable sautéed, steamed, or grilled and mixed with other approved vegetables- use herbs of choice

| | | |
|---|---|---|
| Weight | Bbt | Water day prior |
| Hrs slept | Stress level 1-10 | |
| Menu switches | | |
| Exercise- intensity/duration | | |
| Health- symptoms | | |
| Digestion | | |

## Day Thirteen: No test, any approved protein

### Breakfast
Flax with approved fruit

### Lunch
Salad with leftover vegetables and almond slivers
Carrot soup with sunflower seeds

### Snack
Katie's Kale Chips
Or
Zucchini noush

### Dinner
Approved protein
Mixed greens with radicchio or frisée and avocado, pumpkin seeds
Vegetables of choice grilled, steamed or sautéed-

| | | |
|---|---|---|
| Weight | Bbt | Water day prior |
| Hrs slept | Stress level 1-10 | |
| Menu switches | | |
| Exercise- intensity/duration | | |
| Health- symptoms | | |
| Digestion | | |

## Day Fourteen: Optional bread test

### Breakfast

Any approved breakfast
Or
Bread with almond butter, ½ piece approved fruit

### Lunch

Leftover vegetables on a bed of baby romaine with pumpkin seeds
Basil escarole soup with chia seeds

### Snack

1 oz salt free potato chips
Or
Apple chips

### Dinner

Approved protein on a bed of baby romaine or frisée with avocado, sunflower seeds
Roasted, Sautéed or Grilled Vegetables that have been approved

| | | |
|---|---|---|
| Weight | Bbt | Water day prior |
| Hrs slept | Stress level 1-10 | |
| Menu switches | | |
| Exercise- intensity/duration | | |
| Health- symptoms | | |
| Digestion | | |

## Day Fifteen: No test, any approved protein

### Breakfast
Blueberry Pear Compote
Or
Approved tested Cereal with 2 tbsp chia seeds, 2 tbsp sunflower seeds and approved fruit

### Lunch
Approved Salad with 15 grams of vegetarian protein (no rice)—*see list at beginning of menus for vegetarian protein options*

### Snack
Katie's Kale Chips
Or
12-15 almonds

### Dinner
Any approved protein
Warm Kale Salad
Baby romaine with frisée or radicchio with grated carrot and pear

| | | |
|---|---|---|
| Weight | Bbt | Water day prior |
| Hrs slept | Stress level 1-10 | |
| Menu switches | | |
| Exercise- intensity/duration | | |
| Health- symptoms | | |
| Digestion | | |

## Day Sixteen: Optional test new vegetable

### Breakfast
Blueberry Pear Compote
Or
Approved Cereal with 2 tbsp chia and 2 tbsp sunflower seeds with approved fruit

### Lunch
Leftover Kale with pumpkin seeds, goat cheese
Optional: basil escarole soup

### Snack
Carrots with 2-3 tbsp hummus (if you have tested chickpeas) or almond butter
Or
Zucchini noush

### Dinner
Approved protein on a bed of baby romaine
Steamed, grilled or sautéed approved vegetables
Radicchio with grated carrot
Optional: Add new vegetable to test with dinner

| | | |
|---|---|---|
| Weight | Bbt | Water day prior |
| Hrs slept | Stress level 1-10 | |
| Menu switches | | |
| Exercise- intensity/duration | | |
| Health- symptoms | | |
| Digestion | | |

## Day Seventeen: No test, any approved protein

### Breakfast

Flax granola

Or

New Cereal with chia seeds, sunflower seeds and approved fruit

### Lunch

Leftover dinner vegetables (reheated) on a bed of baby romaine with 2 tbsp hemp seeds and pumpkin seeds

Optional: basil escarole soup

### Snack

Trail mix (almonds or roasted pumpkin seeds and a handful of raisins)

Or

Carrots or 1 Rye crackers with raw almond butter or hummus (only if you have tested)

### Dinner

Approved protein on a bed of baby romaine or frisée

1 cup Vegetable Timbale

Optional- add new vegetable

| | | |
|---|---|---|
| Weight | Bbt | Water day prior |
| Hrs slept | Stress level 1-10 | |
| Menu switches | | |
| Exercise- intensity/duration | | |
| Health- symptoms | | |
| Digestion | | |

## Day Eighteen: Test new vegetable or new restaurant

### Breakfast

New Cereal with chia seeds, sunflower seeds and approved fruit
Or
Approved Breakfast

### Lunch

Baby Romaine with 2 cups vegetable timbale (reheated) and pumpkin seeds
½ apple or pear

### Snack

1 oz potato chips with 1/8th cup homemade guacamole

### Dinner

Test restaurant
Or
Approved protein on a bed of baby romaine or frisée
Test new vegetable sautéed, steamed, or grilled and mixed with other approved vegetables- use herbs of choice

| | | |
|---|---|---|
| Weight | Bbt | Water day prior |
| Hrs slept | Stress level 1-10 | |
| Menu switches | | |
| Exercise- intensity/duration | | |
| Health- symptoms | | |
| Digestion | | |

**Day Nineteen: No test**

Repeat favorite day thus far with most weight loss

| | | |
|---|---|---|
| Weight | Bbt | Water day prior |
| Hrs slept | Stress level 1-10 | |
| Menu switches | | |
| Exercise- intensity/duration | | |
| Health- symptoms | | |
| Digestion | | |

**Day Twenty: No Test**

Repeat favorite day thus far with most weight loss

| | | |
|---|---|---|
| Weight | Bbt | Water day prior |
| Hrs slept | Stress level 1-10 | |
| Menu switches | | |
| Exercise- intensity/duration | | |
| Health- symptoms | | |
| Digestion | | |

## Five Day Menu- Women

**<u>Good Low Reactive Sources of Protein</u>: Aim for 15 grams of protein for lunch unless you are an athlete and then go for 25 grams.**

**Broccoli** — 5 grams per cup (good source of calcium!)
**Sunflower seeds** —5 grams per oz (good source of calcium!)
**Pumpkin seeds** —9 grams per oz (great source of zinc for your immune system!)
**Almonds** — 8 grams per oz
**Cheese** — 8 grams per oz
**Chickpeas** —5 grams per 1/2 cup
**Rice** — 6 grams per 1 cup
**Chia** —5 grams per 2 tbsp (A great source of omega-3's!)
**Hemp Seed** — 11 grams per 3 tbsp (great for iron, magnesium, potassium and zinc)
**Kale** – 6 grams per 1.5 cups

**Portions** — All the portions we use on the plan are the least reactive amounts. If you would like to use larger portions please test them first.

**Natural Sugars** — Most people do well with moderating their intake of natural sugars such as fruit, sweet potatoes, carrot ginger soup and winter squashes. Roasted vegetables fall into this category as well, as the natural sugars are increased when cooked for a long period of time. Find your own balance by starting off with 1.5 servings fruit daily, orange veggies no more than 1x per day and roasted veggies twice a week. You can test a higher frequency or amount of these as you would like.

**Please HYDRATE!** Your baseline is half your body weight in ounces — the best way to do this is drink a pint all at once and please be finished by 7:30 or 3-4 hours before bed. Please do not drink over this amount, this will affect kidney function and will cause water retention.

**Dense Food Guidelines**

- 1 dense grain carbohydrate a day MAX (rice or bread)
- 1 animal protein a day MAX
- 1 bean a day MAX

*If you want to try more than one serving of these per day you can plug a larger portion in for a test day!*

**Combination Tests**

Combining animal protein, grain or legumes together at the same meal is a test. Example: rice (grain) and fish (animal protein) or bread (grain) and eggs (animal protein).

**NOTE**: In winter we always have either a cooked vegetable or a soup with lunch to aid digestion. Dinner always has cooked vegetables and a raw vegetables salad as raw vegetables contain enzymes.

# Time to get started!

1. Create a list of all the foods that have worked for you in the table below.
2. Create a list of foods that are mildly inflammatory and please limit their usage to once every 7-10 day and always follow with a friendly day.
3. Retest all foods that tested as inflammatory in 3-6 months. You may be able to reduce sensitivity to this food and have on occasion, always follow with a friendly day.

| Friendly Foods | Mildly Inflammatory Foods (limit to once every 7-10 days) | Inflammatory Foods (omit for 3-6 months) and re-test |
|---|---|---|
| | | |

## Day 1 (No test)

*Using the outline below, create a menu using your friendly foods.*

**Breakfast — 10-40 grams of protein**

**Your Breakfast:** ________________________________

**Lunch 15-25 grams of protein**

Create a lunch with 15 grams of protein
*In winter add a soup or cooked vegetable to enhance digestion*

**Your Lunch**:________________________________

**Snack**

**Your Snack**: ________________________________

**Dinner 25-60 grams of protein**

Approved protein, Approved Salad, Approved cooked vegetables

**Your Dinner**:________________________________

| | | |
|---|---|---|
| Weight | Bbt | Water day prior |
| Hrs slept | Stress level 1-10 | |
| Menu switches | | |
| Exercise- intensity/duration | | |

## Day 2 (Test Exercise)

*Using the outline below, create a friendly menu (or use your favorite friendly day thus far) but test exercise as the new variable.*

**Breakfast 10-40 grams of protein**

**Your Breakfast**:

______________________________________

**Lunch 15-25 grams of protein**
In winter add a soup or cooked vegetable to enhance digestion
**Your Lunch:**

______________________________________

**Snack**

______________________________________

**Dinner 25-60 grams of protein**
Approved protein, Salad, Approved cooked vegetables

**Your Dinner**:

______________________________________

| | | |
|---|---|---|
| Weight | Bbt | Water day prior |
| Hrs slept | Stress level 1-10 | |
| Menu switches | | |
| Exercise- intensity/duration | | |

## Day 3 (No test)

*Follow the guidelines to create another friendly menu. Follow protein guidelines, this is crucial for success! Remember to limit all portions to recommended portions until larger portions are tested.*

**Breakfast 10-40 grams of protein**

____________________________________________

**Lunch 15-25 grams of protein**

____________________________________________

**Snack**

____________________________________________

**Dinner 25-60 grams of protein**

____________________________________________

| | | |
|---|---|---|
| Weight | Bbt | Water day prior |
| Hrs slept | Stress level 1-10 | |
| Menu switches | | |
| Exercise- intensity/duration | | |

## Day 4 (Test new breakfast item)

*Using the outline below, create a friendly menu but test a new breakfast item. Ideas are whole or lactose free milk, eggs or a new fruit.*

**Breakfast 10-40 grams of protein**

______________________________

**Lunch- 15-25 grams of protein**

In winter add a soup or cooked vegetable to enhance digestion

______________________________

**Snack**

______________________________

**Dinner 25-60 grams of protein**

Approved protein, Approved salad, Approved cooked vegetables

______________________________

| | | |
|---|---|---|
| Weight | Bbt | Water day prior |
| Hrs slept | Stress level 1-10 | |
| Menu switches | | |
| Exercise- intensity/duration | | |
| Health- symptoms | | |

## Day 5 (No test)

*Follow the guidelines of Day 1 to create another friendly menu.*

**Breakfast 10-40 grams of protein**

________________________________________

**Lunch 15-25 grams of protein**

________________________________________

**Snack**

________________________________________

**Dinner 25-60 grams of protein**

________________________________________

| | | |
|---|---|---|
| Weight | Bbt | Water day prior |
| Hrs slept | Stress level 1-10 | |
| Menu switches | | |
| Exercise- intensity/duration | | |

# Recipes

## Apple Cumin Chips

- 2 medium Granny Smith Apples
- 2 tsp cumin
- fresh black pepper, dash sea salt

Preheat oven to 200 degrees

Place half of cumin mix on parchment paper or nonstick pan

Slice apple thin place half on cumin- sprinkle top with remaining

Bake 90 min until crisp- immediately peel and let cool- keeps for 1 week in airtight container

## Apple Streusel

*Streusel Topping*

- 1 ½ cup almond flour
- 1/8th cup brown sugar
- 1 tsp cinnamon
- ¼ cup butter, room temp

*Apple Filling*

- 3 apples, cored and chopped into 1/2 inch pieces
- 1/8th cup brown sugar
- 1 tsp cinnamon
- ½ tsp cardamom
- ¼ tsp cloves
- 4 eight oz. baking ramekins

Preheat oven to 350.

In a small bowl mix all ingredients for streusel topping by hand or with hand mixer.

In a medium bowl combine all apple filling ingredients and mix well. Add apple mixture to mason jars and pack down with ½ inch of streusel topping.

Bake for 25-30 minutes until streusel topping is lightly browned. Serve warm or refrigerate.

**Apricot Glaze (spicy)**

- ½ cup Apricot Jam
- ¼ - ½ cup water
- Chipotle in Adobo Sauce- 1 tbsp.
- Option 2- smoked chipotle powder – 2 tsp (less sodium) available at Fairway

**Basil Escarole Soup**

- 1 large white onion, fine diced
- 1/8th cup dried basil
- 1/2 tsp pink Himalayan sea salt
- 1 tsp black pepper
- 1/4 cup evo
- 1 liter low sodium vegetable stock
- 1 liter water
- 1 tsp agave or honey
- 2 lbs. carrots, chopped
- 8 cups zucchini pasta or 8 cups chopped zucchini, small
- 2 heads escarole, chopped

In a large soup pot sauté onion and basil in evo. Add sea salt and black pepper and let simmer for 20 minutes. Add liquids, carrots and zucchini and let simmer for 20 minutes.

Add chopped escarole and let simmer an additional 10 minutes. Top with lemon or lime juice.

**Blueberry Pear Compote**

*(Makes 2 servings)*

- 1 cup blueberries
- 1 ripe pear
- ¼ cups water (for extra yumminess you can use Silk coco milk instead! Can do ¾ c water and ¾ c coco milk)
- ½ cup chia seeds
- ⅛ cup almond slivers (omit if reactive to almonds)
- 1 tbsp. agave
- Cinnamon to taste- suggested ½ tsp can add cardamom, nutmeg, cloves too (all great digestives)

Chop the blueberries and pear and let simmer for 8-10 minutes in a pot of water (or coco milk) with cinnamon and agave. Remove pot from heat and add chia seeds, and stir frequently for 2 minutes – stir 1 more minute and then let sit in refrigerator for at least 4 hours before serving.

Can be served cold or warm. To warm, microwave for 30 seconds or add to heated coco milk or rice dream. Top each serving with almonds.

**Carrot Beet Salad**

Grate 4-5 carrots and 1 small beet. Should make 4 servings- stores well in Tupperware.

## Carrot Ginger Soup

This recipe, updated from The Plan, is for making the soup in bulk.

1 Tbsp cinnamon
1 Tbsp cumin
1 Tbsp freshly ground black pepper
1 tsp cloves
1 tsp cardamom
½ tsp turmeric
½ tsp allspice
2 Tbsp extra-virgin olive oil
7 quarts water
5 lbs carrots, chopped
2 large red onions, chopped
3 large zucchini, chopped
8 cloves of garlic, peeled
5–6 inches of ginger, peeled

Add the cinnamon, cumin, black pepper, cloves, cardamom, turmeric, and allspice to a dry skillet and sauté, stirring constantly for 30 seconds. Add 7 quarts water to large soup pot. Add the carrots, onion, zucchini, garlic, and ginger to the water and then add toasted spices. Bring the water to a boil and then let simmer for 45 minutes until the carrots are soft. Reserve 2 quarts of water for future soup stocks. Blend the carrot soup in batches.

Yield: 5 quarts, about 10–16 servings

**Note:** Add 1 can of full-fat coconut milk and 5–6 Vietnamese chili peppers for a creamier, spicier soup!

**Cream of Broccoli Soup**

*(Makes 6-8 servings)*

- 3 tbsp. butter
- 1 large onion chopped
- ½ tsp celery seed (dried)
- 2 cups low sodium chicken broth
- 2 cups water
- ½ can full-fat coconut milk
- 8 cups broccoli, chopped (about 4 heads of broccoli)
- 4 cups zucchini, chopped (about 2 medium zucchini)
- 1 small to medium avocado
- 1 tbsp. chipotle in adobo sauce (sub Sriracha if you don't have this on hand)
- Ground black pepper to taste
- Add seasonings to taste – cumin, turmeric, cayenne etc.

Sautee onion and spices in 3 tbsp. of butter. Add in coconut milk, water and chicken broth along with the broccoli and zucchini and cook until vegetables are tender.

Add in avocado, blend and serve! For a less creamy soup add more water. Lime or lemon juice to taste.

Serve immediately, or store and refrigerate up to 5 days.

**Flax Granola**

- 1 cup whole flax seeds
- ½ cup water
- cinnamon, nutmeg clove to taste
- Optional pure vanilla extract raisins, walnuts, cranberries, etc. to taste (please be sure to include only nuts you have tested)

Soak 1 cup of flax overnight in the fridge in roughly 1/2 cup of water with cinnamon.
Spread in a thin layer on a baking sheet and bake at 275. Turn several times to dry out.

Optional add raisins and nuts of choice last 10 minutes. Should bake in 50-60 min.

**Indian Spice Rub**

- 6 tbsp. salt free curry powder
- 1/4 tsp sea salt
- crushed red pepper or cayenne
- ground cumin
- ground coriander
- turmeric
- cinnamon
- ground ginger
- 1-2 tbsp. brown sugar

Combine ingredients. The ones that don't have a quantity- use a 6:1 ratio and adjust to taste. Store in airtight container- good for 4-6 months.

**Kale Salad (warm)**

Sauté 5-6 cups of chopped kale with 4 shitakes in EVOO and herbs of choice. This will be your salad base. Let cool and add your favorite topping.

**Katie's Kale Chips**

- 1 bunch kale, chopped
- 1 tbsp. Extra Virgin Olive Oil
- Pinch of salt
- Freshly ground black pepper
- Optional: 1 tbsp. red pepper flakes
- Fresh lime juice

Preheat oven to lowest setting, about 120F. Make sure the kale is dry, the coat lightly in Extra Virgin Olive Oil and add salt, pepper, and chili flakes, if desired. And lime juice at the end. Spread kale on a baking sheet and bake for 40 minutes to 1 hour.

**Orange Zest Oil**

Zest 1 thoroughly washed medium sized lemon or 1 small orange for ½ cup evo (extra virgin olive oil).

If you prefer a more intense oil, use 2 pieces of citrus. As you adapt to a lower sodium diet (recommended guidelines are 1500 mg or less) the use of flavors OTHER than salt enhances more than just taste. You improve your health and vitality Use the citrus oil to drizzle on steamed vegetables, broiled fish or make a flavorful vinaigrette!

**Plan Trail Mix**

- 1/8th cup sunflower seeds
- 1 tbsp. dried cranberries

**Quick Spicy Coco Sauce**

- 1 can coconut milk- do not use low fat please.
- 1 large onion
- 3-4 cloves of garlic
- spices: ginger, cinnamon, cumin, turmeric, black pepper and cayenne
- 1 tbsp. brown sugar

Sauté ginger, cinnamon, cumin, turmeric, garlic, onion, black pepper and cayenne- all to taste. Add ½ tsp salt and 1 heaping tbsp. brown sugar. Reduce for 20 min- will hold for 5 days or can freeze remainder. Portion is 1/8th cup per serving.

**Simple Guacamole**

- 2 ripe avocados
- 1/2 red onion, minced (about 1/2 cup)
- Juice of half a lime
- 1/8th tsp. sea salt
- Fresh black pepper
- Optional: add 1/2 tomato and/or 2 tbsp. cilantro chopped

Cut avocado in half and remove pit. Using a fork, mash the avocado. Add the chopped onion, cilantro, lime, salt and pepper and mash some more. Can add water for creamier texture. Add optional ingredients now.

If not serving immediately keep avocado pit in to prevent guacamole from turning brown and cover.

**Sunflower Tahini**

- 1 cup sunflower seeds
- 1/4 cup extra virgin olive oil
- 1/4 cup water
- 1 garlic clove, peeled
- 2 tbsp. lemon juice
- dash sea salt
- optional: add more water for creamier tahini

Add all ingredients to a food processor and blend until smooth, about 3 minutes.

Serve immediately, or store and refrigerate up to 5 days.

**The Plan Smoothie**

*(Makes 1 serving)*

- 1 ripe pear
- ½ cup berries
- ¼ avocado
- ¼ cup chia
- Rice Dream (RD) or Silk Coconut Milk (SCM)
- Option- 1 tsp honey or agave
- Option- vanilla extract or cinnamon

Fill Blender with enough RD or SCM to fill to 16 or 20 oz.

Blend. Ice is not recommended if you have thyroid dysfunction.

**Tahini-Free Hummus**

- 2 cups drained well-cooked or canned low sodium chickpeas, liquid reserved
- 1/4 cup extra-virgin olive oil, plus oil for drizzling
- 2 cloves garlic, peeled
- Sea Salt and freshly ground black pepper to taste
- 1 tbsp. ground cumin, to taste, plus a sprinkling for garnish
- Juice of 1 lemon
- Chopped fresh parsley leaves for garnish (optional)

Put everything except the parsley in a food processor and begin to process; add the chickpea liquid or water as needed to allow the machine to produce a smooth puree.

Taste and adjust the seasoning (you may want to add more lemon juice).

Serve, drizzled with the olive oil and sprinkled with a bit more cumin and some parsley.

**Timbale**

This is a great dish to keep adding vegetables in as you test them!

- ½ head of kale
- 1 large zucchini
- 1 red onion
- ½ large carrots
- 4-6 oz goat cheese
- 2 oz parmesan or manchego
- 6 shiitakis

Preheat oven to 400 F. Use a mandolin or slice vegetables as thinly as you can. Create layers like a lasagna: zucchini, onions, swiss chard, goat cheese, carrots, shitakes, swiss chard, carrots, zucchini and top with parmesan. Cook for 30 minutes or until top layer of cheese is slightly golden.

**Zucchini-Noush**

*I love babaganoush, but like many of my clients, I am reactive to eggplant. Subbing zucchini was a natural idea with this summer's bounty and thus was born zucchini-noush!*

- 1/4 cup extra virgin olive oil
- 1 large white onion chopped fine (approx 2 cups)
- 1/4 cup cumin
- 1 tbsp. pink Himalayan sea salt
- 1/8 cup water
- 5 large zucchini chopped (approx 10 cups) oil for baking sheet
- optional: 1 cup sunflower tahini

Add oil to a large skillet on medium heat and add onion, cumin and sea salt. Stir until spices are thoroughly mixed and then mix in water. Lower heat to lowest setting and let simmer for 30 minutes stirring often.

Add zucchini to the onion and mix well. Take zucchini/onion mixture and spread on a well-oiled baking sheet. Bake at 325 for 40 minutes.

Remove from zucchini from the oven and add to a medium mixing bowl. Mix well. The zucchini will break down to a chunky texture. Optional, add 1 cup sunflower tahini and mix well.

## Shopping List – Days 1-7

| **Spices and Herbs (fresh and Dried)**<br>***Note: Where optional is indicated you can omit from recipes and just use more cinnamon*** | |
|---|---|
| All Spice | 1 Container-*OPTIONAL* |
| Basil | 1 Container, 1 bunch |
| Black Pepper | 1 Container |
| Cardamom | 1 Container-*OPTIONAL* |
| Cayenne | 1 Container |
| Celery Seed | 1 Container-*OPTIONAL* |
| Chipotle in Adobo sauce or Sriracha sauce | 1 Jar |
| Cinnamon | 1 Container |
| Cloves | 1 Container-*OPTIONAL* |
| Cumin | 1 Container |
| Ginger - Dried | 1 Container |
| Ginger – Fresh | 5-6 inches |
| Italian herb blend | 1 Container |
| Low Sodium Vegetable Broth | 1 Quart (freeze rest) |
| Maine's Sea Seasoning (kelp or dulse varieties) | 1 Container-*OPTIONAL* |
| Mint (fresh) | 1 bunch- OPTIONAL |
| Nutmeg | 1 Container-*OPTIONAL* |
| Olive oil | 1 Bottle |
| Oregano | 1 Container |
| Parsley (fresh) | 1 bunch- OPTIONAL |
| Rosemary | 1 Container |
| Sea Salt | 1 Container |
| Thyme | 1 Container |
| Turmeric | 1 Container |
| Vanilla Extract | 1 Bottle |

| **Nuts and Seeds** | |
|---|---|
| Almond Butter - Raw | 1 Jar |

| | |
|---|---|
| Almond Flour | 1.5 Cups |
| Almond Silvers | 2 Tbsp |
| Almonds | 38 almonds |
| Chia Seeds | 10 Tbsp |
| Flaxseeds | 5 Cups |
| Hemp Seeds | 2 tbsp-OPTIONAL (only if testing) |
| Pumpkin Seeds | 6 Ounces |
| Sunflower seeds | 2 Cups |

| **Fruit and Vegetables**<br>**Note: *Amounts are approximate—you may need up to 1.5x the amounts listed below for fruits and vegetables.*** | |
|---|---|
| Apples | 7 Apples |
| Apples – Chips | *Bare Fruit* Package |
| Avocado | 3 Avocados |
| Blueberries | 4.5 Cups |
| Cranberries (dried) | 2 Tbsp |
| Lemon | 13 Lemons |
| Orange | 1 Orange |
| Pears | 4 Pears |
| Pomegranate Arils | 1/8 cup |
| Beets | 2 Beets |
| Broccoli | 22 Cups (11 heads) |
| Carrots | 8 Pounds |
| Frisée | 4 Cups |
| Garlic | 27 Cloves (4 Bulbs) |
| Kale | 4 Bunches |
| Lettuce – Baby Romaine | 20 Cups |
| Lettuce – Red Leaf | 2 Cups |
| Onion | 9 Large Onions |
| Onion – Red | 2 Large Red Onions |
| Radicchio | 2 Head Radicchio |
| Shitake mushrooms | 11-12 Large |
| Zucchini | 15 Large, 4 Medium |

| **Fish Protein and Dairy Products** | |
|---|---|
| Butter | 1 Pound |
| Goat Cheese | 3 Ounces |
| Manchego Cheese | ½ Ounce |
| Wild white fish, scallops or egg whites | 4-6 Ounces of fish or 3-4 egg whites |

| **Miscellaneous** | |
|---|---|
| Chocolate – with 25% to 65% cocoa | 1-2 Bars |
| Agave | 1 Bottle |
| Apricot Jam | 1 Jar |
| Basmati rice | 1 Package |
| Brown Sugar | 1 Package |
| Chickpeas | 1 can- OPTIONAL (only if testing) |
| Coconut Milk - Full fat | 2 Cans |
| Coffee | 1 Package |
| Honey | 1 Jar |
| Lentils | 1 cup (will need 1-2 more cups more if you pass this test on day 3) |
| Red Wine | 1 Bottle |
| Silk Coconut Beverage or Rice Dream | 2 Quart Carton |

11355170R00043

Printed in Great Britain
by Amazon.co.uk, Ltd.,
Marston Gate.